Back Pain Breakthrough

NOTE FROM THE AUTHOR

I'd like to wish you congratulations for taking your first step. The fact that you're here reading this right now is testament to the fact that you are ready to make a BIG change and find a way to conquer your back pain.

As a husband, father, business owner, CSCS and student physical therapist - I know first-hand how easy it is to get bogged down by life. As a fellow traveler on the path of pain and resilience, I have a personal history with pain and injury. So, I completely understand how scary it can be to struggle to find relief and regain freedom from pain. I have personally been through various systems that failed me. With that said, it means the world to me that you're willing to take a stab in the dark in trying to accomplish what may sometimes feel like the impossible.

It is my promise to you that it IS possible to break free of the cycle of pain. With a little bit of effort, a great plan, and a sprinkle of psychology, you'll be well on your way to making the change that you've been seeking for so long.

My goal is and has always been to be somebody who can help make a great change in people's lives. That change is led by helping people regain their freedom from pain by optimizing movement, functionality, and restoring confidence in the innate resiliency of the human body. So, I'd like to thank you for being kind enough to put your trust in me. and giving me the opportunity to help you.

By picking up this book, it is my hope that you will not only find success along your back pain relief journey, but also obtain the tools that you need to successfully reach your goals.

Yours,

Justin Levinas

PS.

I am the originating success story that was the motivation, not only for writing this book but for sharing this wealth with the world. This book is the culmination of well over a decade of not only being a chronic back pain patient myself, but also over thirty years' worth of research on injury mechanisms and biomechanics of the spine conducted by others. I've spent countless hours reading research, trialing, and failing with various treatment methodologies. Countless hours experimenting with myself as the guinea pig. Ultimately, that has led to my success.

I would never offer something that I haven't tried myself. Putting this information out there for free is testament to my commitment to making a real difference in the lives of those struggling with back pain. I've experienced firsthand the challenges, frustrations, and setbacks that can accompany this journey. But through my own dedication, relentless pursuit of knowledge, and the implementation of effective strategies, I've managed to conquer my back pain and regain a life full of vitality and freedom.

I firmly believe that sharing this wealth of information speaks to my unwavering belief in the potential for change. Every tool, every technique, every piece of advice within these pages is rooted in my own experiences and the transformative power they hold. I am not just an author; I am living proof of the potential for healing and recovery.

My journey was the spark that ignited the creation of this book, but it's the collective potential of all those who will read it that truly fuels my passion. I am evidence that change is possible, and I am committed to guiding you on a path towards that same transformation. With the knowledge, strategies, and stories shared in these pages, you hold the power to rewrite your own success story—one of triumph over pain, resilience in the face of challenges, and a life reclaimed from the shackles of back pain.

Remember, I am here not just as an author, but as a fellow traveler on this journey. I've walked the path, and now I'm here to walk it alongside you. Let's embark on this transformative journey together, armed with knowledge, determination, and the unwavering belief that a pain-free, vibrant life is within your reach.

The only thing I ask of you is to share this book with those who you think can use it and say something nice in a review if this book has helped you. It costs nothing, and it can help get this book in the hands of somebody who may really need it.

<u>**Disclaimer: Not Intended as Medical Advice**</u>

The information presented in this book is provided for educational and informational purposes only. It is not intended to be a substitute for professional medical advice, diagnosis, or treatment. Always seek the advice of your physician or other qualified healthcare provider with any questions you may have regarding a medical condition or treatment options.

The content of this book is based on research, personal experiences, and general knowledge related to the subject matter. However, every individual's situation is unique, and the information provided may not be suitable or applicable to your specific circumstances.

The use of any information contained in this book is at your own risk. The author and publisher disclaim any liability for any injury, damage, or adverse effects arising from the use or application of the information provided.

It is important to consult with a qualified healthcare professional before making any decisions related to your health or well-being. Do not disregard professional medical advice or delay seeking it based on information you have read in this book. If you have a medical emergency, call your healthcare provider or emergency services immediately.

By reading this book, you acknowledge and agree to the terms of this disclaimer.

<u>INTRODUCTION</u>

Let's face it.

If you're reading this page right now, chances are you've made previous attempts to address the chronic pain you're dealing with.

Whether you're frustrated by constant pain and discomfort affecting your well-being and performance...Or you come home feeling pain and stiffness from long hours of desk work... Or maybe you're grappling with the aftermath of a life-changing injury, like I did, wondering if you'll ever live a "normal" life again...

You've put effort into seeking relief. Yet, despite spending your money on treatments and consulting various experts, the relief you desire seems elusive, if it comes at all.

It's time to start being honest with yourself - Your current approach is simply NOT WORKING. The professionals that you've seen mean well. Unfortunately, good intentions alone don't change how your body feels. You might try to ignore the discomfort and just keep moving forward hoping that the pain will just go away.

But those sleepless nights when back pain feels unbearable, or the workouts where you struggle to perform like you used to... they take a toll on you. Not just physically, but mentally and emotionally. With so many unsuccessful attempts and promising solutions falling short, it can feel lonely. You might feel like you're the only one facing this seemingly unsolvable problem.

Ultimately, you're left with two options:

1. Accept chronic pain as your new normal. Deal with the spasms, ending up on the floor for a week or so, every few months when your "back goes out" – wondering if you need to get to the emergency room.
2. OR find a solution that provides lasting relief.

Accepting a life filled with aches, pains, and imbalances doesn't seem like a viable option. So, it's time to embark on a journey to end chronic pain and resolve those issues for good.

In the realm of chronic back pain, life can feel like a relentless battleground. Every move is met with hesitation, every moment is spent thinking of the lurking worry of discomfort. It's a reality that countless individuals, just like you, navigate day in and day out. But here's the revelation that changes the game: you're not powerless. You're not destined to be held hostage by pain.

Nevertheless, I understand what it feels like to have "the system" fail me. I understand what it's like to get my hopes up and be crushed when searching for solutions and finding more pain and more problems. Ultimately, the best person to help you is yourself, but it can be a daunting task to go at it alone. That's what this book is for.

After years of trial and error, spending significant amounts on experts and medical bills, I discovered a proven path to eliminate pain and feel comfortable in my body.

For this approach to work, you must understand how the body functions. Specifically, there are three key things that are crucial to understand:

1. The source of your pain isn't always where it hurts.

2. You need a system to identify where your pain originates to know how to treat it correctly.

3. Lasting relief is possible, but it depends on addressing **the right problems, at the right time, and with the right intensity.**

Understanding these points is crucial in creating an effective solution to chronic pain. To uncover the true cause of your pain, you must look beyond the symptoms themselves. For instance, focusing solely on fixing my sciatic pain after my accident was not enough. It was only when a movement therapist addressed my entire body and found that I had long standing fear of movement, and subsequent weakness in other parts of my body, that I began to find some relief.

Many people experience pain in one area, but the source of the problem lies elsewhere. Each person's situation is unique. Addressing chronic pain effectively requires a systematic approach, spotting hidden pain points that our bodies learn to compensate for over time. Moreover, solving the right problems in the right sequence is vital.

To not make pain any WORSE or create NEW PROBLEMS, the trick is to identify the problems that you currently have, temporarily MODIFY the aggravating factors, then find the proper re-entry point for movement for YOUR body. Once you've laid down those pillars, the last piece of the puzzle is to follow the proper INTENSITY of exercises to make your road to recovery as seamless as possible.

Together, we'll embark on a journey that WILL be transformative, and full of REAL solutions. Your chronic back pain is not a life sentence. It's a challenge—a challenge we're about to conquer, head-on, with resilience and expertise that comes not only from me and my own life experiences, but from within you.

You're not alone in this struggle. In fact, countless individuals just like you are grappling with back pain, day in and day out. And I'm here to tell you that you have the power to rewrite this narrative, to reclaim your life from the burden of pain.

Welcome to a journey that will redefine how you perceive your body, your pain, and your potential. This isn't just another book or program; it's the beginning of your roadmap to freedom. Overcoming back pain isn't reserved for the lucky few. It's within your grasp, and I'm going to show you how to seize it with both hands.

In the pages that follow, we'll navigate through the maze of objections, skepticism, and doubt that might be holding you back. We'll arm you with the knowledge and confidence to treat your own back pain, because you are your own greatest advocate. The tools, strategies, and mindset shift you'll discover here are not just about managing pain—they're about unleashing your full potential and living a life unburdened by discomfort.

It's time to rewrite your story, to reclaim your strength, and to conquer your back pain once and for all. Are you ready to take the first step? Let's dive in.

<u>PART 1 – UNDERSTANDING BACK PAIN AND UNVEILING BACK PAIN MYSTERIES</u>

The Pain Cycle

In the dimly lit room, I sat on the edge of my bed, wincing as I attempted to get my socks on. The familiar ache in my lower back had intensified once again, reminding me of the unrelenting cycle I found myself trapped in.

Each morning, I woke up with a sense of dread, knowing that my back pain would be waiting for me. The simple act of getting out of bed felt like an uphill battle, a struggle against the persistent ache that had become my unwelcome companion. As the day progressed, my movements grew more cautious, my once vibrant energy now restrained by the fear of triggering a flare-up. Simple tasks became Herculean feats as I navigated a minefield of pain.

But what truly defined the cyclical nature of my back pain was the way it seeped into every facet of my life. It wasn't just physical; it was emotional. My confidence wavered as I declined invitations to social events, fearing that my pain would steal the spotlight. I found myself withdrawing from activities I loved, second-guessing my abilities, and mourning the loss of my former self.

The cycle repeated itself: pain led to fear, fear led to avoidance, and avoidance led to isolation. I had become a prisoner of my own body, trapped in a relentless loop that seemed impossible to escape. I'll never forget the day that I asked my father to "please just find somebody to take my leg off, I can't take it anymore." – if only it would make the excruciating traveling sciatic pain go away. It was this all-encompassing cycle that motivated me to seek a way out, to break free from the chains of chronic pain and reclaim the life I once knew. And as I embarked on my journey to healing, I held onto a glimmer of hope—that with the right knowledge, tools, and determination, I could finally break the cycle and emerge stronger, resilient, and pain-free. I just had no idea where to start.

Chronic pain is a cyclical issue and can be a relentless and debilitating journey. It's marked by a series of interconnected factors that can perpetuate and amplify discomfort. It's called **The Pain Cycle**. It usually starts with an initial trigger, such as a sudden injury, muscle strain, or structural issue like a herniated disc. This trigger generates acute pain and alarms your body that something is wrong.

In response to pain, our muscles in the area tense up as the body's natural protective mechanism. This is called muscle tension and guarding and is a natural response meant to prevent further injury. It can also lead to stiffness and restricted movement. The discomfort and tension can alter how you move and can lead to altered movement patterns where you favor certain movements to avoid pain. These are compensatory strategies which can lead to overuse and strain in compensatory areas.

When pain alters movement, you may begin to avoid certain activities or exercise altogether, resulting in deconditioning, reduced joint flexibility, and weakened supporting structures. Over time, the fear of triggering pain can develop. This is called 'fear avoidance' and can further limit movement.

The cumulative impact of altered movement mechanics, muscle tension, compensatory strategies and fear avoidance can lead to a loss of normal function and range of motion. This cycle continues and takes a toll on mental well-being. Frustration, anxiety, or even depression are common emotional responses to persistent discomfort. These emotions can further amplify the perception of pain through the interplay between mind and body.

Before you know it, you feel like you're falling apart everywhere. Pain pops up in places that you didn't even know hurt you, and you are so confused with everything that's going on that you don't even know what to tell your healthcare provider when they ask what's wrong. **Does this sound familiar?**

Our goal is to put a fork in the pain cycle and break free from chronic pain. This requires a multifaceted approach to address not only the physical, but the psychological and lifestyle factors that are involved in the pain cycle. We interrupt the cycle by gradually reducing pain, restoring function, and building confidence in our ability to move.

Exploring Common Causes and Triggers of Back Pain

Your back plays a vital role in your body's movements, providing the ability to move, support and stability. Yet, as life unfolds, various factors can disrupt this harmony, leading to the unwelcome intrusion of back pain. Let's go over some of the most common causes and triggers that set the stage for this discomfort, shedding some light on the culprits that may be hiding in plain sight.

1. Sedentary Lifestyle – Modern life often involves long hours of sitting, whether at a desk, in front of a screen, or during commutes. This sedentary lifestyle can weaken core muscles, strain spinal discs, and contribute to poor posture. The hunched shoulders and rounded back that result from prolonged sitting can exert pressure on spinal structures, setting the stage for pain to come about.

2. Overuse and Repetitive strain - Repetitive motions or activities that strain the back **when our bodies aren't**

ready for such movements — such as spinal flexion under load — can lead to muscle fatigue, microtrauma, and damage to your vertebrae and discs. Over time, this wear and tear can result in chronic pain, especially if we never take a step back to recondition our bodies to be ready for those motions.

3. Poor Ergonomics - The environments we spend time in can contribute significantly to back pain. Incorrectly set up workstations, poorly designed chairs, and awkward positions can strain your spine and muscles. Whether it's the height of your computer screen, the placement of your keyboard, or the lumbar support of your chair, small adjustments can make a big difference in reducing discomfort.

4. Sleeping Position – We spend roughly a third of our lives asleep. Assuming poor positions while we rest for hours at a time can be problematic for your back. It can also be your best friend.

5. Age-Related Changes – As we age, the natural wear and tear on our discs and joints might contribute to back pain.

6. Poor Posture – Slouching or maintaining poor posture for extended periods of time can strain muscles, ligaments, and discs in the back, leading to discomfort. This doesn't mean that you need to stand at attention like a navy seal

24/7. However, your next posture is your best posture. Variability is key.

These are just a few of the most common causes of back pain. But simply understanding these common triggers can empower you to make more informed choices about your daily activities, movements, and lifestyle habits. You can take proactive steps to prevent or alleviate back pain. In the following chapters, I'm going to help you build a strategy to do just that.

This Issues with Current Low Back Disorder Treatment Practices

I'll never forget the first time that I sought help from the medical world. I was recommended to a pain management specialist who delivered news that felt like a life sentence. "Unfortunately," the doctor said in his solemn tone, "you'll likely be in pain for the rest of your life."

His words hung heavily in the air, casting a shadow over my hopes for a pain-free future. To cope with the chronic pain, he prescribed an arsenal of pain pills. I left his office with a bag full of prescriptions and a heavy heart. I was a 17-year-old kid.

Desperate for relief, I explored alternative therapies and stumbled upon chiropractors. Eager for anything that promised relief, I gave it a try. The first adjustment was like a roller coaster ride for my spine, but not in a good way. The pain intensified, as if my body was protesting the sudden twists and turns. Despite my initial optimism, after another couple of sessions, I quickly realized that chiropractic care was not the magical solution I had hoped for.

Disheartened but not defeated, I sought the guidance of physical therapists, hoping they would have the expertise to ease my suffering. However, my encounters with these therapists left much to be desired. It seemed they followed a one-size-fits-all approach to treatment. "Three sets of 10 reps" were the magic words that echoed in every session, a cookie-cutter solution that they prescribed to everyone with back pain.

Weeks turned into months, and I grew weary of the repetitive exercises that offered no real relief. My frustration deepened as I yearned for a therapist who truly understood the complexities of my back disorder. Each session felt like a ritual, devoid of progress or understanding.

Over time, my pain began to recede. It wasn't a miraculous overnight transformation, but a slow, steady journey toward healing. It taught me that sometimes, the medical system's one-size-fits-all solutions may not be the answer. As I look back on my tumultuous journey, I realize that I didn't need prescriptions, cookie-cutter exercises, or quick fixes. **What I needed was**

resilience, determination, and the courage to carve my own path towards recovery.

You see, many clinicians, physical therapists and chiropractors included, are simply not competent when it comes to dealing with the complicated nature of back disorders. If you've been given a cookie cutter routine that didn't work, it's typically because there is rarely ever a one-size-fits-all when it comes to lower back disorders. There is no single method of treatment that will work for everybody, yet it's all too commonly seen in clinics.

The truth is, most clinicians either simply don't understand the intricacies, or have not personally dealt with the physical and mental war that chronic back pain can be Most family doctors will admit that they don't know what to do with back pain patients. They're trained to prescribe medications. Medication that simply dulls your pain usually only makes matters worse, as you continue to contribute to aberrant movement patterns, or avoid moving altogether while simply numbing the symptoms.

Yes, we all learn the basics through schooling, but spine related issues often require a very different approach than what is typically taught in school. For example, the rudimentary approach to rehabilitation is to identify what is weak and then strengthen it. Or identify where it hurts and work on it. Chronic back pain often requires a different philosophy that includes more than just manual techniques and exercise.

While we are all humans and share some fundamental movement patterns, recognize that we all have unique anatomy and therefore will require a unique approach that is tailored to our own specific needs. In the pages that follow, we will explore various methods to sit, stand, walk, lift, sleep, think, and live pain free. Be mindful of the fact that **you will have to experiment** to find what works best for you.

Debunking Myths and Misconceptions to Demystify Your Back Pain

Back pain is a topic that's surrounded by a multitude of myths and misconceptions. These misconceptions often lead to confusion, unnecessary fear, and ineffective approaches to managing and preventing back pain. Let's debunk some of the most prevalent myths and set the record straight:

Myth 1: Rest is the Best Solution – While rest is important during the acute phase of an injury, prolonged bed rest can actually weaken muscles and delay recovery. Staying active with appropriate exercises and movements is crucial for promoting healing and preventing further issues.

Myth 2: Back Pain Equals Serious Damage – Experiencing back pain doesn't necessarily mean there's serious damage to your spine. In many cases, pain is a result of muscle strain, tension, or minor issues that can be managed with the right tools.

Myth 3: Only Older People Get Back Pain – Back pain doesn't discriminate based on age. People of all ages can experience back pain due to various factors. Interestingly, most people have less back pain around the age of retirement and its younger folks that are most affected.

Myth 4: Pain Equals the Need for Surgery – Abraham Maslow once said, "I suppose it is tempting, if the only tool you have is a hammer, to treat everything as if it were a nail." Surgeons assume that everything can be fixed with a scalpel, if only you give them a chance to cut the pain out of you. The fact of the matter is that the tissues being targeted for removal are rarely the only cause of pain. Risks associated with surgery very often don't outweigh the potential benefits. Surgery should be considered as a LAST resort. Most back pain can be managed through non-invasive methods like exercise, physical therapy, a sprinkle of psychology and lifestyle changes. You simply need to find the right approach or combination of approaches.

Myth 5: Bed Firmness Matters Most – While mattress support is important, there's no one-size-fits-all solution. The ideal mattress firmness varies based on individual preferences and body types. A mattress that provides support and comfort is key.

Myth 6: All Exercises Are Off-Limits – In reality, the right exercises can be extremely beneficial for back pain. In fact, exercise is likely going to be your best friend throughout this journey. Avoiding all physical activity is NOT the answer. The key is finding the RIGHT entry exercises for YOU.

Myth 7: Back Pain is All in Your Head – Back pain is a real physical sensation. While stress and emotions can contribute to pain, pain itself is not solely a psychological issue.

Myth 8: You Should Avoid Bending and Lifting – Proper lifting techniques and movements are important, and trying to avoid bending and lifting altogether is not only an extremely difficult task, but it will also hinder your ability to perform daily activities. While it may seem like a scary thought, we don't want to avoid bending or lifting at all. We just want to be a little more conscious of HOW we bend or lift. While those movements may seem difficult now, there are MANY regressions that can prepare us for being able to perform them without causing further pain or any damage. Once again, it's about finding the right entry point for YOU, then progressing appropriately. More on this later.

Myth 9: Heat or Ice are Always the Best for Pain Relief – While heat can provide temporary relief for muscle tension, it's not always the best solution. Cold therapy can be more effective during the acute phase of an injury to reduce inflammation. Ultimately, neither of these are long-term solutions.

Myth 10: You Can't Prevent Back Pain – While some factors are beyond our control, adopting a healthy lifestyle, staying active, and practicing proper body mechanics can significantly reduce the risk of developing back pain. Just about everybody gets some back pain at some point or another. But just like understanding potential triggers of back pain, by gaining some clarity on myths and misconceptions, you'll be better equipped to make informed decisions about your back health and seek out strategies that are tried, true and effective.

Myth 11: Back pain is hereditary – Back pain is not a life sentence, and you aren't destined to have it. Your pain is not written in stone. While genetics do make some people more susceptible to back issues, it's something that can be treated and often avoided altogether.

Myth 12: My MRI will give the doctors everything they need to know for treating me – Determining the cause of pain from an MRI is like trying to understand why a computer isn't working just by looking at its external casing. While MRIs and CT scans CAN be useful, they are just a small piece of evidence to build a case for you. They do NOT, however, tell the full story. MRIs or CTs are very limited in what they can tell us. They might show changes or certain features that may or may not be the source of your pain. Much more commonly, how we move (or more importantly how we don't), our activity levels, our lifestyle choices, and how we think influence our pain levels more than the diagnoses we receive from our MRI results.

I will use myself as an example here. My MRI results stated that I had disc herniations all throughout my lumbar spine that were pushing on my sciatic nerve on my LEFT side. If the results of my MRI correlated properly with the pain I was feeling, I'd have been in a lot of pain on my left side – right? Well, all the pain that I was feeling was on my right. So those results became a good coaster for my morning coffee. Don't let MRI results scare you and understand that those findings may just be incidental. The correlation between what an MRI says and what you are actually feeling is quite poor.

Myth 13: I can "desensitize" myself to back pain by just working through the pain – For some strange reason, a common theme when people are in pain has become to move INTO pain thinking that you will desensitize yourself to it. I get it. Mobility training has become the new thing, and everybody wants to be able to turn themselves into a pretzel. There's also the old mantra "no pain, no gain". But unfortunately, this does not always apply. Let me ask you this. If you smash your face into a wall, will it hurt less every subsequent smash? Obviously not. When you have chronic back pain, moving into that pain will only make you more apprehensive to additional movement. The best way to start finding relief is to stop smashing your face into the wall. That is – find what movements cause your back pain, then REMOVE them from the equation by finding alternative strategies. The secret is in changing your movement patterns so that you can enjoy exercise instead of fearing it. At first, this can be daunting. With time and practice, it gets easier.

Myth 14: Yoga and Pilates are great ways to alleviate back pain – Yoga and/or Pilates are very often recommended to those with back pain. While these may be beneficial to some, they can be detrimental to others. There are components of both yoga and Pilates that can actually aggravate the pain of people with certain back conditions. Ultimately, there is NO SUCH THING as a single program that is a one-sized-fits-all. That's why it's so important to figure out what is right for you, and that's what we're here for.

Myth 15: Stretching will reduce my back pain – Just like Yoga or Pilates, there is no such thing as a stretch that is good for all patients. Every person is different, and every person's body is different. Stretching stimulates the "stretch reflex" which reduces pain sensitivity and provides about 10-20 minutes of pain relief for some. However, there are others who need to shorten their muscles to restore a proper length-tension relationship. When they don't, this ends up creating a cycle where you constantly feel the need to "stretch it out" to get some relief, not realizing that you may be contributing to your pain. The focus should instead be on figuring out whether stretching is beneficial for YOU, and progress based on your assessment instead of guesses.

Myth 16: I just need to make my muscles stronger to fix my back pain – Dr. Stuart McGill said "Think about strength in relation to your body like horsepower in relation to a car. If a souped-up 500-hoursepower engine is put inside of a dinky, broken down car and then raced at top speed, it's only a matter of time before the mega-engine rips the frail frame and suspension to pieces". Maintaining proper movement patterns requires muscular strength, but equally importantly – muscular endurance. For that reason, rehabbing a spinal condition will often require us to place endurance at an equal priority to strength. Ultimately, we need to establish a subtle balance between strength, power, endurance, and mobility – not simply focus on strength alone.

Part 2: Overcoming Objections and Building Confidence

As I faced the daunting journey of self-treatment for chronic back pain, I encountered some of the most stubborn barriers and objections that tried to keep me trapped in the cycle of discomfort. The biggest challenge was the lack of knowledge. I realized that I had been living in the dark about the underlying causes of my pain, making it nearly impossible to choose the right treatments. Doubt and confusion clouded my decisions, leaving me feeling lost in a sea of options that promised relief but often delivered disappointment.

Incorrect form during exercises was another major hurdle. I vividly recall the frustration that came with realizing that my well-intentioned efforts were exacerbating the issue. Overambitious workouts further fueled my setbacks. Impatient for rapid results, I pushed my body beyond its limits, only to experience setbacks that plunged me back into the grip of pain. And let's not forget the nagging fear that my efforts would trigger more pain. This fear, like a persistent shadow, whispered doubts in my mind every time I considered attempting exercises or movements that could potentially worsen the situation.

Despite these challenges, I pressed forward, driven by a deep desire to find a solution. It was a journey filled with trial and error, and even moments of doubt. However, overcoming each barrier and objection was a testament to my resilience and determination. I discovered that with the right guidance, patience, and the willingness to adapt my approach, I could overcome these obstacles and pave the way to a life free from chronic back pain.

In my experience, the biggest problems and objections with self-treatment are listed below. Fortunately, I have already dealt with these issues. Therefore, along with those issues, I will explain how I will help you navigate them so you can leave the guesswork out.

Objection 1 – Fear of Making it Worse – It's a valid concern—fear of taking the wrong step and aggravating the pain further. This book includes simple instructions on where to start to meet yourself where you currently are. You're about to learn how to examine the various components of your training (or lack thereof) and translate it into the art of targeted, effective self-treatment. No more uncertainty. No more tiptoeing around. You will learn to assess your pain triggers and revamp your aggravating activities to actually reduce your pain.

Objection 2 – Lack of Knowledge – Ignorance about back pain and its solutions can be paralyzing. We're flipping the script. We will dive into understanding your body, its intricacies, and the powerful tools you can use to conquer pain.

Objection 3 – Belief in Professional Expertise – This is valid reasoning - professionals have their place, and good ones can help you expedite your journey to relief. It's always a good thing to have trained eyes helping you. Finding a good physical therapist that understands and directly addresses the cause of your pain is amazing. But they are few and far between. Nevertheless, educating yourself and being proactive in your own treatment can pay dividends.

Objection 4 – Preference for Quick Fixes – Quick fixes often lead to temporary relief – if that. You're done with that cycle. What you'll find here are not band-aids, but strategies and gameplans to rewrite the narrative of your relationship with pain. In a world that craves instant gratification, patience is a virtue. The journey is a marathon, not a sprint. Each step is a note of progress, and with persistence, your relief will set in.

Objection 5 – Perceived Complexity – The labyrinth of back pain can seem impenetrable. I am handing you a compass—a roadmap that breaks down the complex into actionable steps, ensuring you never feel lost again. In a sea of advice, clarity is a rarity. I will help you navigate the ocean of information by providing a simple-to-follow guide to relief.

Objection 6 – Misconceptions – Misconceptions can mislead you on your journey, causing unnecessary fear and worry. That is exactly why we went through debunking the various myths that may plague you on your journey to recovery. With this book in your possession, you will always have that chapter to look back at should any doubt be sewn into your mind.

Objection 7 – Past Failed Attempts – Previous attempts that fell short don't define your journey. If you feel like you've tried everything, I've been there. The truth is, if something didn't work for you, then it wasn't the right solution. Consider this your reboot, your fresh start armed with knowledge, tools, and a roadmap for lasting relief.

Objection 8 – Fear of Commitment – Commitment can be daunting, especially when you may have tried and failed in the past. But here's the beauty: the commitment we're talking about is to your own well-being. Trial and error are part of the challenge, and this is the path that is achievable and sustainable.

Objection 9 – Desiring Professional Validation – You're not alone in seeking validation, and I am easily reachable for help. But what if you could validate yourself? With every small victory over pain, you'll know that you're on the right track.

Objection 10 – Ignoring Lifestyle Factors – Imagine addressing not just the pain, but the very factors that fuel it. Poor posture, sedentary habits, and sleepless nights are the threads we'll untangle.

Objection 11 – Failure to Address Underlying Imbalances – Underneath your pain lies a plethora of imbalances that are waiting to be harmonized. I will guide you to unraveling the mess of pain that you are feeling.

Objection 12 – Unrealistic expectations – Relief isn't an overnight fix, it's a journey of progress. You will learn to set realistic expectations and recognize and embrace each step forward.

Now that you have a solid foundation with respect to the most common myths, misconceptions, and objections to self-treatment, let's explore the benefits.

The beauty of this program is four-fold.

Firstly, self-treatment allows you to tailor your approach based on YOUR specific needs. You can explore the options while choosing exercises, and evaluating the lifestyle changes that will most appropriately resonate with you and your body.

Second, self-treatment methods require minimal cost when compared to conventional treatment. This opens the door for so many more people, making it an extremely affordable option for managing and preventing back pain.

Third, long-term results. Since this program is built around your personal needs, you can effectively address the root causes of your pain and are more likely to experience lasting relief. You will be making lifestyle changes here. This will ultimately lead to less and less potential hiccups down the road. Since you can reread this book as many times as you need, it can help you manage those hiccups if they do come along.

Lastly, learning about your body and its needs will help you gain a deep sense of empowerment over your back pain. No longer having to feel confused or helpless, you can actively participate in your own recovery journey.

<u>**Part 3: The Path to Self-Treatment Success**</u>

The Mindset Shift: Embracing a Solution-Oriented Approach

The turning point in my battle against chronic back pain came when I decided to shift from a passive mindset to a proactive, solution-oriented one. For too long, I had been resigned and defeated, feeling like a helpless victim of my own body's limitations. But something inside me snapped, and I realized that I had to find the power to rewrite my story. No longer content with merely enduring the pain, I embarked on a journey of empowerment and self-discovery.

It wasn't an easy transition. The fear of pain and the comfort of the familiar held me back like invisible chains. But with each step I took towards a solution-oriented approach, a new sense of purpose emerged. Instead of dwelling on what I couldn't do, I began focusing on what I could. Seeking guidance and education, I started to understand the intricacies of my body and the sources of my pain. I embraced exercises with correct form, treating each movement as a step towards liberation rather than a chore to endure.

The shift wasn't just physical; it was a mental transformation as well. I shed the limitations I had placed on myself and opened my mind to the possibility of progress. As I saw incremental improvements, my confidence soared, replacing doubt with determination. With a proactive mindset, I no longer feared the pain; I faced it head-on, armed with knowledge, tools, and an unyielding spirit. This shift marked the beginning of my journey from a passive observer to an active protagonist, and it laid the foundation for a future free from the chains of chronic back pain.

Setting Clear Goals and Expectations

With newfound determination, I delved deeper into my journey of conquering chronic back pain. One of the most pivotal realizations was understanding the paramount importance of **setting clear goals and expectations** for my treatment journey. It was as though I had discovered the compass that would guide me through the uncharted territory ahead.

I realized that without clear goals, I was merely wandering without direction. So, I sat down and defined what success meant to me — not just in terms of pain relief, but in terms of regaining my active lifestyle and reclaiming my joy. These goals became my driving force.

As I experimented with exercises and lifestyle changes, each action was infused with purpose. Every movement was a step towards achieving those defined goals, and every ounce of effort felt purposeful. Instead of passively going through the motions, I was actively engaging with my treatment, armed with the knowledge that each effort was contributing to a bigger picture.

Setting goals went hand in hand with setting clear expectations. I learned to acknowledge that progress wasn't always linear; there were setbacks and plateaus along the way. But armed with the right mindset, I viewed these moments as part of the journey, not roadblocks. With the knowledge that recovery takes time and patience, I embraced the process wholeheartedly, celebrating every small victory as a step closer to my ultimate goals.

The transformation in my approach was remarkable. I was no longer just a passive participant in my recovery; I was an active, goal-driven individual who refused to be defined by my pain. This shift in mindset not only fueled my determination but also provided me with the resilience to persevere through challenges. As I walked this path with clear goals and unwavering expectations, I realized that I was not just overcoming chronic back pain; I was reclaiming my life with a renewed sense of purpose and direction.

STOP AND READ CAREFULLY – READ AND PERFORM THE FOLLOWING EXERCISE

Right now, I want you to take a moment to reflect on your pain. Close your eyes and take a few deep breaths. Reflect – how does your pain affect your daily life, activities, and overall well-being?

Find a pen and paper. Or open the notes app in your phone and write down specific instances where the pain has limited you or caused frustration. Hold onto that.

Now, imagine a pain-free life. Envision yourself moving freely, engaging in activities you love without hesitation. What would that look like for you? Write down your goals in clear, specific terms. For example, "I want to be able to play with my children without discomfort," or "I want to hike again without worrying about pain."

Take each of your goals and break them down into smaller, achievable steps. For instance, if your goal is to hike without pain, a smaller step might be to walk for 2 minutes without pain. Then 5 minutes, 15 minutes, 30 minutes, and so on. These smaller steps make your goals more tangible and manageable. One of my favorite quotes is from Bruce Lee who said "A goal is not always meant to be reached, it often serves simply as something to aim at." We will use these as your targets and milestones along your path.

Acknowledge Potential Setbacks: Recognize that progress isn't always linear. There might be days when your pain feels more pronounced, or you face challenges in sticking to your routine. Write down potential setbacks that you might encounter, such as busy days or moments of discouragement.

Set Realistic Expectations: Reflect on the fact that healing is a gradual process. Realize that setbacks and plateaus are a normal part of any journey. Set realistic expectations by acknowledging that your progress might have ups and downs, but every step counts.

Take your goals and steps and create a visual representation. You can use a calendar, a vision board, or a journal. Mark down the steps you'll take each week and the milestones you hope to achieve.

Celebrate every victory, no matter how small. Whether it's walking an extra block or sitting comfortably for longer periods, acknowledge your progress. Write down your achievements and how they make you feel.

Lastly, remember, this exercise is about defining your goals, then creating a rough-draft roadmap that aligns with your goals and expectations. We'll work on the small steps to get that to that ultimate dream outcome together. However, by breaking down your goals into manageable steps and acknowledging potential challenges, you're setting yourself up for success. As you embark on your journey to alleviate chronic back pain, this exercise will serve as a guide to keep you motivated and focused on your path to recovery.

Part 4: Effective Self-Treatment Strategies

Knowledge is Power: Understanding the Basics of Back Pain Relief

When I found myself amid a battle against chronic back pain the pain seemed to have a life of its own. I felt helpless as it dominated my days. But along my journey to understanding the basics of back pain relief, I quickly realized that knowledge was the key to unlocking the door to a pain-free life.

Arming myself with knowledge was like turning on a light in a dark room. I dove into understanding the anatomy of the back – the intricate network of muscles, ligaments, and bones that worked in harmony to support my body. Learning about the key factors that contribute to back pain gave me a new perspective on why the pain persisted.

With this newfound knowledge, I was no longer in the passenger seat of my painful journey. I could identify the triggers and make informed decisions about my approach to relief. Understanding how certain movements and activities impacted my back allowed me to choose exercises that would target the root causes of my pain.

Allow me to give you a simple overview of what I've learned about chronic back pain.

Imagine your back as a complex puzzle, where each piece plays a crucial role. The muscles around your spine provide stability and support, while the discs cushion and absorb shock. But when you're in pain for whatever reason, it's like throwing the puzzle pieces out of order – the result? Discomfort, pain, and limited mobility. We need to put the puzzle pieces back together.

When you're armed with the proper knowledge as you embark on your back pain relief journey, you'll learn to understand why certain exercises work, why others make you feel crappy, and how to avoid aggravating your pain. With the power of knowledge, you're no longer at the mercy of back pain – you're equipped to take charge of your healing process and pave the way for a pain-free future. So, let's dive into the essentials of back health and explore the factors that will lead you to lasting relief.

Core Concepts – Standards for Back Health

This is arguably one of the most important sections that you will read in this book. If your goal is to manage your current back pain, avoid future episodes, and maximize your potential for your back, there are several standards that you MUST adhere to. These standards will act as your guideline for healing and maintaining a durable back, and a pain-free life.

Standard 1 – Practice healthy back activities EVERY SINGLE DAY – Trying to partake in healthy movement every day will ensure that it becomes a habit. The effects of building this habit will compound, and lead to better overall back health.

Standard 2 – Take the 30,000-foot view – Keeping your eye on the big picture requires that you account for many of the various factors that can influence the health of your back, and the rest of your body. How you sleep, how you eat, the kinds of activities that you do – there must be harmony between your lifestyle factors.

Standard 3 – Modifying the aggravating factors – This is arguably the most important standard to adhere to. You will soon see that there is a clear correlation between the movements that you perform and the pain that you feel. To prepare your spine to withstand the stresses of day-to-day life, we need to modify the factors that aggravate the damaged tissues to allow them to adequately heal. If certain postures or movements cause pain, IDENTIFY THEM AND MODIFY THEM (for the time being). Over time, you will be able to re-expand your pain-free repertoire of activity and rebuild your body's ability to tolerate all sorts of movement.

Standard 4 - Understand that progress is not linear and is ever evolving – In the early stages of your journey, you may find that there are very few activities that you are able to perform pain free. As you progress through this program, your movement capabilities will begin to expand, as will your ability to tolerate those movements for longer periods of time and/or under heavier loads. Through a bit of trial and error, you will find the sweet spot for your body, and build from there. There will be days where you've done too much, and it may cause pain. There will also be days where perhaps you've not done enough (though anything is almost always better than nothing). With time and practice, you will learn to operate below the threshold of what causes you pain and find that sweet spot that leads to steady progress.

Finding Your Pain Triggers

A big part of being successful in getting rid of your back pain will be attributed to **finding and modifying the movement behaviors that cause your pain**. To find and know these movements is to know how to find alternative strategies.

Keep in mind, the goal for this program is NOT to simply avoid movement. Afterall, motion is lotion. While you will eventually be able to return to the style of training of your choosing, the goal here is to adopt pain-free, alternative movement strategies while giving you the freedom to start moving again. In addition, we are also reconditioning your brain and nervous system to feel safe during movement instead of feeling threatened and tensing up.

Exercise and Muscular Endurance

While the addition of heavier strength training is reserved for the later stages of rehab, **Exercise and Muscular Endurance** are the two pillars that will not only help you alleviate your pain over time, but also allow you to take control over your body's well-being. You don't need to be a fitness guru or be able to perform insane mobility feats to reap the benefits. In the pages that follow, we will break down each concept into manageable steps, so whether you're a beginner or have been on this journey for a while, you'll find practical strategies that align with your comfort level.

A common question that arises is "why not strengthen the weak links? Wouldn't that help with the pain?". My answer is an analogy that Dr. Stuart McGill used which makes a whole lot of sense. If you take a 500 Horsepower engine, and put it in a rinky-dink beat-up frame, how long before that frame breaks down? One mile? Ten miles? Who knows… The bottom line is that strength without endurance is like horsepower without a solid frame. If you are somebody that has pain with simple, everyday activities like standing or sitting – we need to scale things way, way down and retrain our foundation before we start adding additional load. I'd prefer the 200-horsepower engine that will get me to my destination, rather than the 500-horsepower engine that can break down at any moment.

To relate this to your day-to-day life, you're not utilizing your one-rep-max strength when you're simply walking around, sitting down in a chair, or grocery shopping. When adopting new movement techniques, performing them repeatedly will require a degree of muscular endurance. That is why I prefer to train endurance first.

Some Perspective Before Your Self-Assessment

Let's recap. So far, you have:

1. Learned about the pain cycle.
2. Explored common causes of back pain.
3. Debunked myths and misconceptions.
4. Addressed objections to self-treatment.
5. Learned how to adopt a solution-oriented approach.
6. Learned how to set realistic goals and expectations.
7. Acquired some basics of back pain relief.
8. Learned about the standards for back health.
9. Discovered that finding your pain triggers is of utmost importance.
10. Learned that we need to modify your movements and add some muscular endurance to your repertoire.

You've already come a LONG way in a short time. I'd venture to say that you ALREADY know more than 95% of people when it comes to back pain.

We've established that repeated irritation via painful movements will generally make matters worse. Now it's time to learn how to identify the movements that cause this irritation. This section will guide you through the process of identifying the movements that exacerbate your pain. **I highly suggest that you read this chapter in its entirety with a notebook and pen to record some findings.** So, without further ado, let's get started!

First and foremost, this assessment assumes that there are no serious underlying causes for your pain. It's crucial that your primary care physician (PCP) conducts a comprehensive examination before you engage in any exercise routines. After receiving clearance from your PCP, you can move forward. The goal is to pinpoint the root causes of your discomfort and then tackle them accordingly.

What is typically taught in terms of orthopedic exams is to check spinal range of motion, conduct neurological exams, and measures of strength and reflexes. Many doctors will simply look at an MRI or CT and diagnose the issue with that alone. Physical exams typically last only a few minutes. There is generally a disconnect between what is normally assessed and what helps to reduce current pain.

To reduce the pain that you're currently feeling, the first thing we need to do is identify the most probable cause of your pain. We

will accomplish this by administering provocation tests. That is –
we are going to provoke the pain to the best of our ability to
determine which postures and motions exacerbate your pain, and
which ones offer pain-free alternatives. Once we have a good idea
of what causes your pain, we'll know how to treat it. Now, let's
give you the proper assessment that you deserve.

<u>**PART 5 – YOUR SELF ASSESSMENT AND FIXING THE PROBLEM**</u>

Your Self-Assessment

STEP 1 – It's time to use that notebook and pen that you grabbed earlier.

- Create two columns.
- On the left, write down every activity that you've noticed increases your back pain.
- On the right, write down every activity that you've noticed DOES NOT increase your back pain, and those that you can perform pain-free, if any.
- Now look at the two lists side-by-side and see if you can identify a common factor. Is there a specific posture or movement among the activities that cause pain? Likewise, is there a specific posture of movement that relieves your pain?
- For example, you may find that slouching hurts a lot more than arching your back. Maybe putting your socks on is extremely difficult. But you find that arching your back or laying on your belly are pain free, and maybe even help relieve pain. In this specific case, the pain is posture-related – specifically a flexed spine. We call this "flexion intolerance".   More on that in a bit.

STEP 2 – Necessary questions that you MUST ask yourself.

1. **What makes your pain worse?** Bending forward, sitting for long periods of time, standing for long periods of time, walking, running, squatting with weight on your back, etc. If you can identify any specific activity that triggers your pain, then congratulations! You've officially identified a specific trigger. The next step is to learn how to manage that trigger by adjusting your movement patterns, such that you eliminate the trigger for the time being. Eventually, you will work back up to being able to do those things again. But for now, let's just find out what they are and put them on the back burner for a bit.

2. **Do you ever notice that your pain intensity changes?** If you've noticed that you have pain free intervals and painful intervals, it's worth noting that there is probably a good reason for that. That tells us that there may be triggering postures or movements that you utilize throughout the day. Identifying the triggers will ensure your success in eliminating them.

3. **Does that pain increase throughout the day?** Finding that your pain intensifies as the day progresses indicates that the cumulative loading of your back throughout the day has exceeded your back's current capacity to withstand the stresses that you're placing on it. In essence, you're lacking

muscular endurance somewhere. As we continue to load our backs past our threshold, the pain will increase until you rest. The solution here is to give yourself necessary breaks, and…. You guessed it – improve muscular endurance. We'll cover this shortly.

4. **Does your pain radiate into your butt, legs, and/or feet?** This pain is characteristic of a trapped nerve root in the lumbar spine. It's usually made worse with postural changes such as spinal flexion (bending forward at the spine), for example. Adopting better movement mechanics for our bodies, such that we can modify those painful positions, will help to rid ourselves of the pain.

5. **How does walking affect your pain levels?** Simply walking can give us a lot of information about the type of pain that you're experiencing. Pay attention to the 'type' of walking that you are performing. Many of us are given advice to walk slowly to reduce our pain. But often, walking slowly is more difficult and painful than walking quickly. As we walk slowly, we tend to not use much arm swing, and statically load our spines more than we do when walking fast. On the other hand, when walking quickly we utilize the spring action of our muscles, we tend to use a more upright posture, and generally utilize healthier walking patterns. If all walking is painful, you may just be particularly sensitive

right now. Once you're a bit further along in the program, you will be able to make walking a therapeutic activity. (More on this later.)

STEP 3 – IDENTIFYING TRIGGERS

To pinpoint the cause of your pain, we'll administer provocation tests, provoking the pain to understand which postures and motions worsen it. This will guide us in suggesting movement modifications for pain-free strategies. Keep in mind that it's OKAY if multiple positions exacerbate your pain. Now, let's begin the testing.

TESTS:

1. **Slump Test:**
   a. *Position 1:* Sit in a chair, grab the underside, and slouch. Observe and record your sensations.
   b. *Position 2:* While slouching, tuck your chin down and record any changes in pain. Then extend your neck by looking up. Did this relieve the pain? Record your findings.
   c. *Position 3:* While slouching with your chin tucked, extend one leg out slowly, keeping toes pulled up. Note any changes in sensation in your foot, legs, or back. Repeat

with the other leg.

d. *Note:* Pain may occur at any point during this test.

2. **Extension Compression Test:**

   - Arch your back while seated, pull up on the chair, and note what you feel.

3. **Seated Compression Test:**

   - Sit up tall on the edge of a chair. Do not arch your back or slouch. Grab the underside of the chair and pull up to compress the spine while maintaining an upright posture. If you find this painful, record it.

4. **Heel Drop Test:**

   - While standing, rise onto your toes, then quickly drop your heels back down onto the ground, creating a sudden impact force through your legs and spine. Pay attention to any pain, discomfort, or sensations that you experience during or immediately after the heel drop.

   - Repeat this test again with your chin tucked down toward your chest.

   - Repeat this test again with your neck extended (looking up).

5. **Load Intolerance:**

- Hold the weight at roughly waist height. Pay attention to whether you feel any pain here. If this is comfortable, next you will extend your arms out in front of you while holding that weight. Is this painful? Record your findings.

STEP 4 – ANALYZING RESULTS

1. Pain during the Seated Compression or Heel Drop Test indicates spinal compression as a likely trigger of your pain.

2. **Slump Test Analysis:**

a. Pain in Position 1 suggests posture-related pain. Spinal flexion hurts you and you'll want to modify that for the time being. (more on this later)

b. Pain in Position 2 or 3, especially along the course of the sciatic nerve (Down the back of your leg and sometimes into the foot and pinky toe), suggests a nerve-related component.

3. Pain during the Extension Compression Test suggests spinal extension as a trigger.

4. Pain during the Load Intolerance Test indicates your back is currently load intolerant, meaning placing forces through your spine triggers pain.

STEP 5 – ACCELERATING RECOVERY

Pain-Relieving Positions:

Now that we understand what positions cause your pain, we'll explore pain-relieving positions.

1. **For Compression-Triggered Pain:**

   - Redo the Seated Compression or Heel Drop Test but brace your core before applying compression.

   - Stiffen your core as if somebody is about to punch you in the stomach, then repeat the test. If bracing your core reduces the pain, you've found a tactic to increase your resilience to activities that compress your spine. Now, this doesn't mean you need to walk around with a braced core all day long, but it does give you an idea of where you might start your muscular endurance training. (Hint: it's your core.)

2. **For Slump Test-Triggered Pain:**

   - Start standing, note your pain level, then transition to laying on your belly.

   - Take your time getting into this position, do it slowly and carefully without flexing your spine. First get into a lunge position, then place the front knee down alongside the back knee, then slowly walk your hands down your thighs, onto the floor as you bend through your hips, and finally walk your hands forward so that you're on your hands and knees. Ease into a fully prone position until you're fully on your belly.

- If lying on your belly reduces pain, it is yet another clue which suggests that you are flexion intolerant at the moment. Gentle extension-based exercises like laying on your belly or performing prone press-ups may provide relief during flare-ups.

3. **For Extension-Triggered Pain:**
    - If you've found that the extension-compression test triggered your pain, or that laying on your belly made the pain worse, then you may have pain triggered from extended postures. To confirm, stand up and arch your back while twisting to one side. Do this for both sides. Does this hurt?
    - If one side hurts, stand on one leg (on the same side that you have pain on) and arch your back and twist to that side again. Is the pain less? If so, you have found that stiffening your hips and spine will help to relieve your pain. A "neutral" position is best for you right now.

4. *Finding your Pain-Eliminating Posture:*

- Stand up, face a wall, and place your forearms flat against it, keeping them parallel to each other. Use the wall for support throughout these movements.

- **When performing the following tests, keep in mind that if lumbar motion causes pain, then it may be a trigger for you. You will learn to utilize your hips instead of your spine when performing movements like bending forward or picking things up off the floor for the time being.**

- Hip and Spinal Flexion: Gently hump your hips forward towards the wall as if a string is pulling your hips towards it. It's like you're trying to close the distance between your pubic region and the wall. As you push your hips forward, allow your spine to follow by gently rounding your back as if you're curling into a ball. If this makes pain worse – you've confirmed that flexion is your pain trigger. If it

- Hip and spinal Extension: Now, imagine a string attached to the back of your hips pulling them away from the wall, guiding your hips back as if you're trying to knock something over with your butt. As

- you shift your hips back, let your spine follow by gently arching your back.

- Continue to flow between these movements slowly and deliberately, feeling the gentle stretch and engagement of your muscles with each transition. Explore these movements and find a spine and hip posture that lessens your pain. It doesn't have to eliminate the pain right there and then, but when you find a good balance, it should feel better than before.

- Once you find the right pain-eliminating posture for you, you'll want to incorporate this into as many daily activities as possible. Doing laundry, walking the dog, sitting in a chair, getting up from a chair, etc. Modify these activities to resemble your pain eliminating position as much as possible.

Now that you've tested yourself, assessed your results, and learned about some pain-relieving postures, things should already be a lot clearer for you. You've now identified some of your back pain triggers and learned a handful of techniques about how to alter those movements. Now let's learn about some management techniques and exercises that will help you for the long haul. While there are features of back pain that distinguish one type from another, movement is the medicine that they all need. The caveat is that it must be the right movement and at the right intensity.

THE NON-NEGOTIOABLES

If you've made it this far, congratulations. This is the section that will teach you how to make your daily activities pain free. To do so, you need to LIVE by the top 6 things REQUIRED to repair your spinal injuries. We'll dive into each of them, but here's the list.

1. **Modify the causes of pain and find your pain free postures.**
2. **Develop new movement patterns that allow you to be pain-free or close to it.**
3. **Perform the non-negotiable exercises that help ANYBODY with back pain.**
4. **Keep your hips and T spine mobile.**
5. **Motion is lotion – take on therapeutic walking.**
6. **Practice this list every damn day.**

Modifying the Causes of Pain and Developing New Movement Patterns

So, the first step to modifying the causes of your pain entails identifying your pain triggers. We've just done that in the last section. Now we need to take that information and use it to our advantage to modify those movements that hurt and turn them into easier to manage regressed versions of those very same movements. The goal here is to transform movements that cause pain into more manageable versions, without losing their essence. Think of it as fine-tuning your daily actions to work in harmony with your body, rather than against it.

Here are some examples of everyday movements that you might want to utilize regressions for if you're in pain.

1. Sitting and Standing:

- **Original Movement:** Plopping down into a chair or standing up quickly.

- **Regressed Version:** Approach sitting and standing with control. When sitting, gently lower yourself into the chair, engaging your core and using your leg strength. When standing, do so gradually, pushing through your heels and using your legs and glutes to push yourself up off the chair.

2. Bending Over:

- **Original Movement:** Bending at your lower back to pick something up.

- **Regressed Version:** Bend at the knees and hips, as if you're performing a squat. This method distributes the load more evenly and reduces strain on your lower back. In some instances, this might be painful too. You might consider lunging or reverse lunging while keeping your spine neutral.

3. Reaching for Objects:

- **Original Movement:** Extending arms far out in front of you.

- **Regressed Version:** Keep items at a closer distance and start with smaller reaches. Engage your core and use your leg strength to support the movement. Increase the distance over time as pain decreases.

4. Working at a Desk:

- **Original Movement:** Sitting in the same position for prolonged periods.

- **Regressed Version:** Introduce dynamic sitting. Adjust your position regularly, use an ergonomic chair, and take short breaks every hour to stand, stretch, or walk.

5. Climbing Stairs:

- **Original Movement:** Taking stairs quickly or with poor posture.

- **Regressed Version:** Take stairs one at a time, focusing on your posture. Step fully onto each step, engaging your leg muscles.

Naturally, these examples are simplistic, and it would be impossible to cover every movement regression out there. This is where you might need a bit of help from a pro, but it is also where you have the opportunity to get creative. Your goal here is to find what works for you at this very moment instead of avoiding movement all together. If doing a full squat hurts, you can squat to a chair instead. If bending forward hurts, stay within pain free ranges of motion and progress to larger ranges very slowly. If your back pain gets worse throughout the day, try implementing some static core strengthening by bracing your core, increasing the number of reps or duration of the brace over time.

Start small. Pick one or two movements that you've identified as triggers. Focus on them and gradually incorporate these changes into your daily routine. Over time, these small adjustments can lead to significant improvements in pain management and overall mobility. Slowly but surely, you'll find that your freedom of movement is returning.

Remember, the key is not to avoid movement but to modify it in a way that respects your body's current limitations and strengths. It's about working smarter, not harder, to achieve a pain-free and active lifestyle.

Perform the non-negotiable exercises that can help ANYBODY with back pain.

After lots of trial and error, in my extensive experience both being a patient and in working with individuals suffering from back pain, I've identified a set of exercises that are not only effective but also safe for beginners or those experiencing significant discomfort. These exercises are carefully selected to ensure they can be performed even when you're in a lot of pain, providing relief and promoting recovery. The beauty of these exercises lies in their adaptability; whether you're a novice or further along in your journey to wellness, they can be tailored to your current ability level. The number of repetitions, the duration of each exercise, and the number of sets can all be adjusted according to where you are right now. Over time, you'll want to track your progress, gradually increasing reps, sets, or hold times, as this will be a clear indicator of your improvement and increased strength. Remember, the key is consistent, gradual progress, ensuring a safe and effective path to alleviating back pain.

Exercise 1: Gentle Cat-Camel

Purpose: To relax and mobilize the spine.

Instructions:

1. **Starting Position:** Begin on your hands and knees, with your wrists directly under your shoulders and your knees under your hips.

2. **Cat Phase:** Exhale and gently round your spine towards the ceiling, like a cat stretching. Tuck your chin towards your chest.

3. **Camel Phase:** Inhale and let your stomach drop towards the floor, arching your back. Lift your head and tailbone towards the ceiling.

4. **Movement:** Alternate between the cat and camel positions slowly and smoothly.

5. **Duration:** Perform this for 1-2 minutes, focusing on gentle, fluid, deliberate movements and spending time taking slow deep inhalations and exhalations as you flow from the cat phase to the camel phase.

Exercise 2: The McGill Big 3

Purpose: To build safe core endurance.

a. Curl-Up:

1. Lie on your back with one leg straight and the other bent at the knee.

2. Place your hands under the small of your back for support.

3. Lift your head and shoulders slightly off the ground, keeping your neck in a neutral position.

4. As you lift, brace your core

5. Hold for a few seconds, then lower back down. Repeat for 1 set of 4-6 reps, 10 second holds per rep. Increase the number of sets as you progress.

b. Side Plank:

1. Lie on your side, propped up on your elbow, legs stacked.

2. Lift your hips off the ground, forming a straight line from your ankles to your shoulders. If this is too difficult, you can keep your knees on the ground while lifting your hips up off the ground.

3. Hold the position for a few seconds, then lower down. Do this for 1 set of 4-6 reps, 10 second holds per rep. Repeat on the other side. Increase the number of sets as you progress.

c. Bird-Dog:

1. Start on your hands and knees.

2. Extend one arm forward and the opposite leg back, keeping your back straight.

3. Hold for a few seconds, then return to the starting position. Do this for 1 set of 10 reps before switching to the opposite arm and leg. Be sure to perform these reps slow and controlled.

4. To progress this exercise, you can hold the extended position and "draw squares" with your arm and leg before lowering down and repeating on the other side.

Exercise 3: Resisted Clam Shells

Purpose: To strengthen the hip abductors.

Instructions:

1. Lie on your side with your hips and knees bent at 45 degrees, legs stacked.

2. Place a resistance band around your thighs just above your knees. Keep it light to start.

3. Keeping your feet together, raise your upper knee as high as you can without allowing your top hip to shift backwards. We want to keep the hips stacked.

4. Hold for a moment, then slowly lower back down.

5. Perform 2-3 sets of 10-15 repetitions before switching sides.

Exercise 4: Ball Squeezes

Purpose: For adductor strengthening.

Instructions:

1. Sit or lie with your knees bent and a soft ball between your knees.

2. Squeeze the ball with your knees, engaging your inner thigh muscles.

3. Hold the squeeze for a few seconds, then release.

4. Repeat for 2-3 sets of 4-6 reps, 10 second holds.

Optional Exercises

1. Lunges:

- Great for strengthening glutes and quads, easy on the back.

- Stand with feet hip-width apart.

- Step forward with one foot and lower your hips until both knees are bent at about a 90-degree angle.

- Make sure your front knee is directly above your ankle.

- Push back up to the starting position. Repeat on the other side.

2. Prone Press-Ups:

- Beneficial for those dealing with sciatic pain.

- Lie on your stomach with your hands placed under your shoulders.

- Gently press your upper body up, extending your arms while keeping your hips and pelvis in contact with the floor.

- Hold for a few seconds, then lower back down.

- Safe and effective path to alleviating back pain.

3. Standing Rows:

Purpose: To improve posture by strengthening the upper back muscles.

Instructions:

1. Stand facing a cable machine or resistance band anchored at chest level.

2. Grasp the handles or band with both hands, arms extended, and palms facing each other.

3. Keeping your back straight and core engaged, pull the handles or band towards your torso, squeezing your shoulder blades together.

4. Slowly return to the starting position and repeat.

4. Pallof Press:

Purpose: To strengthen the core, particularly the obliques, and enhance overall stability of the spine.

Instructions:

1. Starting Position: Stand perpendicular to a cable machine or a resistance band anchored at chest height. If using a band, stand far enough away to create tension.

2. Holding the Handle: Grasp the cable or band handle with both hands and hold it against your chest. Ensure your feet are shoulder-width apart.

3. The Press: Slowly extend your arms forward, straight out from your chest, while keeping them aligned with the middle of your chest. Your body will want to twist towards the band or cable, but resist this motion.

4. Hold and Return: Hold the extended position for a moment, then slowly bring your hands back to your chest.

5. Repetition: Perform several repetitions before switching sides to face the opposite direction.

Keep your hips and Thoracic spine mobile!

Lower back pain is often a symptom of limited mobility in other areas of the body, particularly the hips and thoracic spine (upper back). When these areas lack flexibility and range of motion, the lower back compensates by taking on extra work and movement, leading to strain and discomfort. Incorporating gentle mobility exercises for the hips and thoracic spine can significantly alleviate this stress on the lower back. Here's how these exercises help and some examples to include in your routine:

1. Hip Mobility Exercises:

- **Hip Circles:**

    - Stand and hold onto a chair or table for support.

    - Lift one leg and rotate the hip in large, circular motions, both clockwise and counterclockwise.

    - Repeat on the other side.

- **Pigeon Pose (Modified):**

    - Sit on the floor with one leg bent in front of you and the other extended behind.

    - Gently lean forward over the bent leg, feeling a stretch in the hip.

    - Hold for 30 seconds and switch sides.

2. Thoracic Spine Mobility Exercises:

- **Thoracic Extensions on a Foam Roller:**

    - Lie back on a foam roller placed under your upper back.

    - Support your head with your hands and gently arch over the roller.

- Move the roller up and down your upper back, pausing at tight spots.

- **Open Books**

  - Lie on your side with support for your head and neck

  - Open the Book: Keeping your knees together and pressed to the floor, lift your top arm and open it out to the other side, as if you're opening a book. Rotate your upper body as you do this but keep your lower body stationary.

  - Follow with Your Gaze: Turn your head to follow your moving hand.

  - Make sure your top hip does not move backwards as you rotate.

  - Take deep breaths as you continue to rotate, feeling a stretch across your upper back.

  - Return to the starting position and repeat for 5-10 repetitions. Turn over and repeat on the other side.

Motion is Lotion – Take on Therapeutic Walking.

Understanding Therapeutic Walking

Therapeutic walking involves more than just a casual stroll. It's a mindful, structured approach to walking that focuses on posture, pace, and technique to specifically target and alleviate back pain.

Key Components of Therapeutic Walking:

1. Posture: Maintaining a good posture is crucial. Keep your head up, shoulders back, and spine in a neutral position.

2. Stride: Opt for shorter, more controlled strides to reduce the impact on your back.

3. Pace: Start with a slow to moderate pace and gradually increase as your comfort allows.

4. Breathing: Practice deep, rhythmic breathing to help relax your muscles and improve oxygen flow.

Implementing a Walking Regimen

1. Start Slow: Begin with short walks, gradually increasing the duration as your endurance improves.

2. Consistency: Aim for regular walks, ideally daily, to reap the most benefits.

3. Mindful Walking: Be conscious of your body, posture, and movements during your walk.

4. Comfortable Footwear: Wear supportive shoes that provide good cushioning and arch support.

Overcoming Challenges

- Pain Management: If walking initially increases your pain, reduce the duration and slowly build up your tolerance.

- Weather and Environment: In bad weather, consider walking indoors on a treadmill.

- Motivation: Walking with a friend or listening to music or audiobooks can make the activity more enjoyable.

Therapeutic walking is a simple yet powerful tool in the management of chronic back pain. It's a low-impact, accessible form of exercise that not only addresses the physical aspects of back pain but also contributes to overall mental and emotional well-being. If this is not accessible to you yet, DON'T WORRY – you will get there. For now, focus on what you CAN do instead of what you cannot.

LAST BUT CERTAINLY NOT LEAST... Practice this list EVERY. DAMN. DAY.

PART 6: RECLAIMING YOUR ACTIVE LIFESTYLE

Imagine standing at the base of a mountain, looking up at the peak. You've already climbed so far, surpassing obstacles, and discovering strengths you never knew you had. Now, it's time to take it to the next level and beyond.

You've embarked on a remarkable journey, one that began with the challenge of chronic back pain and has led you here. This final chapter is not just a conclusion, but rather a new beginning. It's about taking everything you've learned and experienced and stepping confidently into a future where pain doesn't dictate your limits.

The road ahead is filled with obstacles, but also possibilities. You've learned how to listen to your body, respect its limits, and gently push them. This isn't just about managing pain; it's about thriving beyond it. Your active lifestyle awaits, filled with the adventures and joys you deserve.

As we close this book, I want to extend my heartfelt thanks to you for embarking on this journey with me. Your commitment to reclaiming your active lifestyle is not just inspiring; it's a beacon of hope for many who are still finding their way, and it's the very motivation for me to continue doing what I do.

I am rooting for you every step of the way. Your journey doesn't end here – it evolves. The strategies and insights you've gained are tools that will continue to serve you as you explore new horizons.

This book is just the beginning. There's more to explore, more to learn, and more ways to grow. I look forward to expanding on this content to bring you so much more for you build on what you've learned and take you even further.

If you ever find yourself needing guidance or support, know that I am here. You are a welcomed resident of a community that understands your journey, your hardships, and celebrates your victories.

Embrace your active lifestyle with joy and confidence. You've earned every moment of it. Here's to your health, your happiness, and your unending journey of discovery and growth.

Cheers,

Justin